CORONARY ARTERY DISEASE: Causes, Symptoms, Diagnosis, Treatment and Prevention

By

Kurt G. Martinez

Table of contents

INTRODUCTION

Coronary artery disease (CAD, also called coronary heart disease, or CHD) is caused by the narrowing of the large blood vessels that supply the heart with oxygen. These are called coronary arteries. Arteries that have become extremely narrow can cause shortness of breath and chest pain during physical activity. If a coronary artery suddenly becomes completely blocked, it can result in a heart attack.

CAD can also lead to other health problems like heart failure or heart rhythm problems. Various treatments can be used to reduce the symptoms and the risk of complications.

Chapter 1: Causes of Coronary Heart Disease

Coronary illness (CHD) is typically brought about by a development of greasy stores (atheroma) on the walls of the corridors around the heart (coronary supply routes).

The development of atheroma makes the supply routes smaller, confining the progression of blood to the heart muscle. This cycle is called atherosclerosis.

Your gamble of creating atherosclerosis is altogether expanded if you:

smoke
have hypertension (hypertension)

have elevated cholesterol
have elevated degrees of lipoprotein (a)
try not to work-out consistently
have diabetes
Other gamble factors for creating atherosclerosis include:
Being large or overweight
having a family background of CHD - the gamble is expanded in the event that you have a male relative younger than 55, or a female relative under 65, with CHD

Smoking
Smoking is a significant gambling factor for coronary illness. Both nicotine and carbon monoxide (from the smoke) put a burden on the heart by making it work quicker. They likewise

increment your gamble of blood clumps.

Different synthetics in tobacco smoke can harm the covering of your coronary corridors, prompting furring of the supply routes. Smoking essentially expands your gamble of creating coronary illness.

Hypertension
Hypertension (hypertension) overwhelms your heart and can prompt CHD.

Elevated cholesterol
Cholesterol is a fat made by the liver from the soaked fat in your eating regimen. It's fundamental for sound

cells, however a lot in the blood can prompt CHD.

Peruse more about elevated cholesterol.

High lipoprotein (a)

Like cholesterol, lipoprotein (a), otherwise called LP(a), is a kind of fat made by the liver. It's a realized gamble factor for cardiovascular infection and atherosclerosis.

The degree of LP(a) in your blood is acquired from your folks. It's not regularly estimated, yet screening is suggested for individuals with a moderate or high gamble of creating cardiovascular sickness.

Absence of ordinary activity

Assuming you're latent, greasy stores can develop in your supply routes.

Assuming that the corridors that supply blood to your heart become obstructed, it can prompt a coronary failure. Assuming that the conduits that supply blood to your cerebrum are impacted it can cause a stroke.

Diabetes

A high glucose level might prompt diabetes, which can over two times your gamble of creating CHD.

Diabetes can prompt CHD in light of the fact that it might make the covering of veins become thicker, which can confine blood stream.

Apoplexy

An apoplexy is a blood coagulation in a vein or conduit.

In the event that an apoplexy is created in a coronary course it forestalls the blood supply from arriving at the heart muscle. This normally prompts respiratory failure.

Chapter 2: Symptoms of Coronary Heart

What are the side effects of coronary supply route infection?

Track down a heart subject matter expert.

You might have coronary supply route infection (computer aided design) and not even know it. Coronary supply route infection happens when your coronary corridors, the veins that convey blood to your heart, are restricted or become obstructed.

Coronary supply route sickness happens in light of the fact that a greasy substance called plaque develops in your coronary corridors. The plaque development can prompt supply route limiting and inevitable solidifying, which confines blood stream to your heart. Fortunately, some way of life changes and prescriptions can help you delay or forestall coronary illness. At Aurora Medical services, our cardiologists give full-range care to forestall or treat coronary supply route infection.

Early indications of coronary supply route infection

Many individuals have no coronary supply route infection side effects from the beginning. Be that as it may, as plaque development deteriorates, you might insight:

Chest torment (angina)

Heart palpitations, which might feel like a hustling or beating heartbeat

Windedness, particularly when you endeavor

Some of the time, the principal indication of coronary supply route infection is a cardiovascular failure. As a matter of fact, coronary supply route infection is one of the most widely recognized reasons for cardiovascular failures. A cardiovascular failure is a health related crisis that requires prompt treatment. On the off chance that you believe you're having a cardiovascular failure, call 911 right away.

Normal cardiovascular failure side effects

A cardiovascular failure is an unexpected blockage of blood supply to your heart. It's essential to perceive the indications of a cardiovascular failure so you know when to call for crisis help for yourself or a friend or family member.

Cardiovascular failure side effects can fluctuate, however the most widely recognized side effects include:

Chest torment, particularly on the left side or focal point of your chest
Inconvenience that transmits from your chest through your shoulders or arms
Jaw, neck or back torment
Sensations of completion, tension or pressing in your chest
Windedness, even very still

Shortcoming or discombobulation

Indications of a cardiovascular failure in ladies

While ladies may likewise encounter chest torment with a cardiovascular failure, they are more probable than men to encounter subtler coronary episode side effects. These include:

Nervousness

Back torment

Trouble resting

Acid reflux

Queasiness

Extreme exhaustion

Since these side effects might be less unexpected or explicit, numerous ladies postpone looking for treatment for a cardiovascular failure. Be that as it may, the sooner you seek treatment for a cardiovascular failure, the less harm your heart muscle maintains. On the off chance that you experience any cardiovascular failure side effects, look for crisis care right away.

Normal coronary supply route infection side effects

The side effects of coronary supply route infection can fluctuate from one individual to another, however many individuals experience:

Chest torment

Exhaustion

Heart arrhythmias (unpredictable heart rhythms)

Heart palpitations

Acid reflux

Windedness

Expanding in the feet or hands

Coronary supply route infection side effects can likewise fluctuate among people. Like cardiovascular failures, coronary supply route sickness side effects in ladies might be more unpretentious than in men. Ladies are bound to encounter jaw torment, windedness or consuming sensations in their chest.

Chapter 3: Diagnosis of Coronary Heart Disease

To analyze coronary supply route infection, a medical care supplier will look at you. You'll probably be asked inquiries about your clinical history and any side effects. Blood tests are normally finished to really look at your general wellbeing.

Tests

Test to help analyze or screen coronary vein infection include:

Electrocardiogram (ECG or EKG): This simple and easy test estimates the electrical action of the heart. It can show how quick or slow the heart is thumping. Your supplier can see signal examples to decide whether you're having or had a respiratory failure.

Echocardiogram: This test utilizes sound waves to make photos of the pulsating heart. An echocardiogram can show how blood travels through the heart and heart valves.
Portions of the heart that move feebly might be brought about by an absence of oxygen or a cardiovascular failure. This might be an indication of coronary vein sickness or different circumstances.

Practice pressure test: On the off chance that signs and side effects happen most frequently during exercise, your supplier might request that you stroll on a treadmill or ride an exercise bike during an ECG. On the off chance that an echocardiogram is finished while you do these activities, the test is known as a pressure reverberation. On the off chance that you can't work out, you may be given meds that invigorate the heart like activity does.

Atomic pressure test: This test is like an activity stress test yet adds pictures to the ECG accounts. An atomic pressure test shows how blood moves to the heart muscle very still and during stress. A radioactive tracer is given by IV. The tracer assists the heart veins with appearing all the more obviously in pictures.

Heart (cardiovascular) CT examine: A CT sweep of the heart can show calcium stores and blockages in the heart supply routes. Calcium stores can limit the conduits.

At times color is given by IV during this test. The color makes itemized photos of the heart supply routes. On the off chance that color is utilized, the test is known as a CT coronary angiogram.

Cardiovascular catheterization and angiogram: During cardiovascular catheterization, a heart specialist (cardiologist) tenderly embeds an adaptable cylinder (catheter) into a vein, typically in the wrist or crotch. The catheter is delicately directed to the heart. X-beams assist with directing it. Color moves through the catheter. The color assists veins with appearing better on the pictures and diagrams of any blockages.

In the event that you have a course blockage that needs treatment, an inflatable on the tip of the catheter can be expanded to open the corridor. A cross section tube (stent) is commonly used to keep the course open.

Chapter 4: Treatment of Coronary Heart Disease

Treatment

Treatment for coronary corridor illness normally includes way of life changes, for example, not smoking, practicing good eating habits and practicing more. Now and then, drugs and methods are required.

Drugs

There are many medications accessible to treat coronary course illness, including:

Cholesterol drugs. Meds can assist with bringing down awful cholesterol and decrease plaque development in the veins. Such medications incorporate statins, niacin, fibrates and bile corrosive sequestrants.

Anti-inflammatory medicine. Anti-inflammatory medicine diminishes the blood and forestall blood clumps. Day to day low-portion headache medicine treatment might be suggested for the essential avoidance of coronary failure or stroke in certain individuals.

Everyday utilization of anti-inflammatory medicine can make serious side impacts, remembering draining for the stomach and digestive tracts. Try not to begin taking a day to day headache medicine without conversing with your medical services supplier.

Beta blockers. These medications slow the pulse. They additionally lower circulatory strain. On the off chance that you've had a coronary episode, beta blockers might diminish the gamble of future assaults.

Calcium channel blockers. One of these medications might be suggested on the off chance that you can't take beta blockers or beta blockers don't work. Calcium channel blockers can assist with further developing side effects of chest torment.

Angiotensin-changing over chemical (Expert) inhibitors and angiotensin II receptor blockers (ARBs). These medications lower the pulse. They might assist with holding coronary course sickness back from deteriorating.

Dynamite. This medication extends the heart courses. It can help control or alleviate chest torment. Dynamite is accessible as a pill, shower or fix.

Ranolazine. This drug might assist individuals with chest torment (angina). It could be endorsed with or rather than a beta blocker.

Medical procedures or different systems Coronary corridor stent Open spring up discourse box

Coronary corridor sidestep a medical procedure Open spring up discourse box In some cases, medical procedures are expected to fix a hindered supply route. A few choices are:

Coronary angioplasty and stent position. This technique is finished to open obstructed heart veins. It might likewise be called percutaneous coronary intercession (PCI). The heart specialist (cardiologist) directs a slim, adaptable cylinder (catheter) to the restricted piece of the heart supply route. A little inflatable is swelled to assist with broadening the impeded conduit and further develop the bloodstream.

A little wire network tube (stent) might be set in the supply route during angioplasty. The stent assists keep the supply route with opening. It brings down the gamble of the corridor limiting once more. Stents gradually discharge medicine to assist with keeping the veins open.

Coronary conduit sidestep a medical procedure (CABG). A specialist takes a solid vein from one more piece of the body to make another way for blood in the heart. The blood then circumvents the impeded or limited coronary course. CABG is an open-heart medical procedure. It's normally done exclusively in those with many limited heart veins.

Chapter 5: Prevention of Coronary Heart Disease

There are multiple ways you can decrease your gamble of creating coronary illness (CHD, for example, bringing down your circulatory strain and cholesterol levels.

Eat a sound, adjusted diet
A low-fat, high-fiber diet is suggested, which ought to incorporate a lot of new products of the soil (5 partitions every day) and entire grains.

You ought to restrict how much salt you eat to something like 6g (0.2oz) a day as a lot of salt will expand your circulatory strain. 6g of salt is around 1 teaspoonful.

There are 2 sorts of fat: soaked and unsaturated. You ought to keep away from food containing immersed fats, in light of the fact that these will build the degrees of terrible cholesterol in your blood.

Food varieties high in soaked fat include:

meat pies
frankfurters and greasy cuts of meat
margarine
ghee - a kind of spread frequently utilized in Indian cooking
grease
cream
hard cheddar
cakes and rolls

food sources that contain coconut or palm oil

Be that as it may, a fair eating regimen ought to in any case incorporate unsaturated fats, which have been displayed to build levels of good cholesterol and assist with diminishing any blockage in your courses.

Food varieties high in unsaturated fat include:

slick fish

avocados

nuts and seeds

sunflower, rapeseed, olive and vegetable oils

You ought to likewise attempt to keep away from an excess of sugar in your eating regimen, as this can build your possibilities creating diabetes, which is demonstrated to expand your possibilities creating CHD fundamentally.

smart dieting
eating less immersed fat
current realities about sugar
Be all the more genuinely dynamic
Joining a solid eating routine with standard activity is the most effective way of keeping a sound weight. Having a solid weight lessens your possibilities of growing hypertension.

Customary activity will make your heart and blood circulatory framework more proficient, bring down your cholesterol level, and furthermore keep your pulse at a solid level. Practicing routinely decreases your gamble of having a coronary failure. The heart is a muscle and, similar to some other muscle, benefits from working out. A solid heart can siphon more blood around your body with less exertion.

Any oxygen consuming activity, for example, strolling, swimming and moving, makes your heart work harder and keeps it solid.

Keep to a sound weight

A GP or practice medical caretaker can let you know your optimal load corresponding to your level and fabricate. On the other hand, figure out what your weight list (BMI) is by utilizing the BMI mini-computer.

Quit any pretense of smoking

In the event that you smoke, surrendering will lessen your gamble of creating CHD.

Smoking is a significant gambling factor for creating atherosclerosis (furring of the conduits). It additionally causes most instances of coronary apoplexy in individuals younger than 50. Diminish your liquor utilization Assuming that you drink, don't surpass the greatest suggested limits.

people are prompted not to drink in excess of 14 units seven days consistently spread your drinking north of 3 days or more in the event that you drink as much as 14 units every week

Continuously keep away from hitting the bottle hard, as this builds the gamble of a coronary episode.

Monitor your pulse

You can monitor your pulse by eating a solid eating routine low in soaked fat, practicing consistently and, if necessary, taking medication to bring down your circulatory strain.

Your objective circulatory strain ought to be under 140/90mmHg. In the event that you have hypertension, request that a GP check your pulse consistently.

Monitor your diabetes

You have a more prominent possibility of creating CHD in the event that you have diabetes. Being actually dynamic and controlling your weight and circulatory strain will assist with dealing with your glucose level.

Assuming you have diabetes, your objective circulatory strain level ought to be under 130/80mmHg.

Take any endorsed medication
Assuming you have CHD, you might be endorsed medication to assist with alleviating your side effects and stop further issues creating.

In the event that you don't have CHD yet have elevated cholesterol, hypertension or a past filled with family coronary illness, your primary care physician might recommend medication to forestall you creating heart-related issues.

Assuming that you're recommended medication, it's indispensable you take it and follow the right dose. Try not to quit taking your medication without talking with a specialist first, as doing so is probably going to exacerbate your side effects and put your wellbeing in danger.

Conclusion

In conclusion, Coronary Heart Disease is a complex and widespread condition that affects millions of people around the world. Understanding CHD and taking proactive steps to manage risk factors and prevent the disease is crucial for maintaining heart health and reducing the risk of serious complications. This book has provided readers with a comprehensive overview of CHD, including the causes, symptoms, diagnostic and treatment options, and lifestyle changes that can help prevent the disease. By incorporating these strategies into their daily lives, readers can take control of their heart health and live a longer, healthier, and more fulfilling life. Remember, your heart is your most valuable asset, and taking care of it is the key to a happy and healthy future.

www.ingramcontent.com/pod-product-compliance
Lightning Source LLC
Chambersburg PA
CBHW012313240726
48656CB00008B/2663